PICTURE BOOK OF
BIBLE VERSES

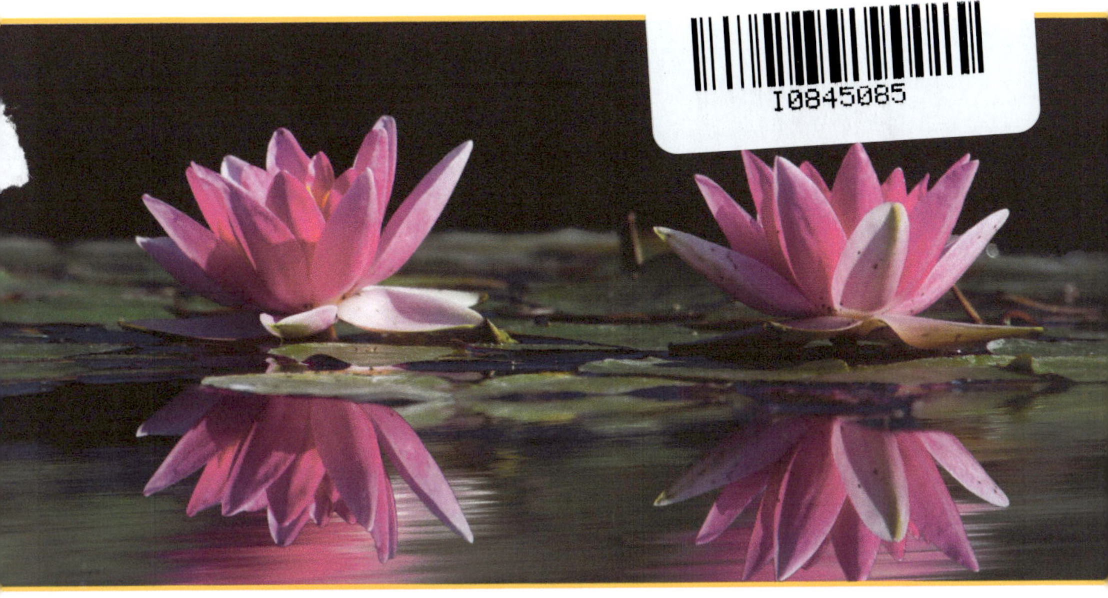

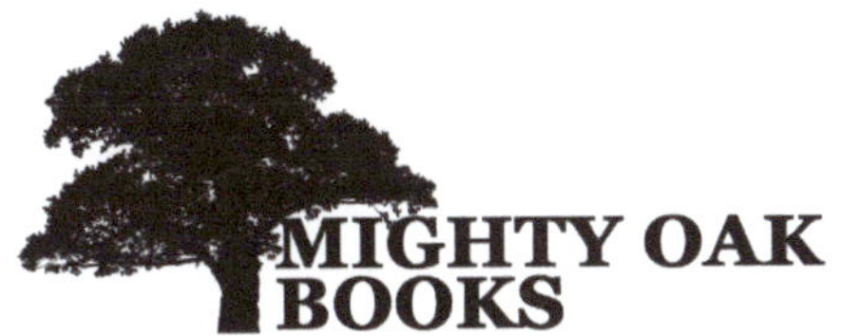

For we walk
by faith,
not by sight.

2 Corinthians 5:7

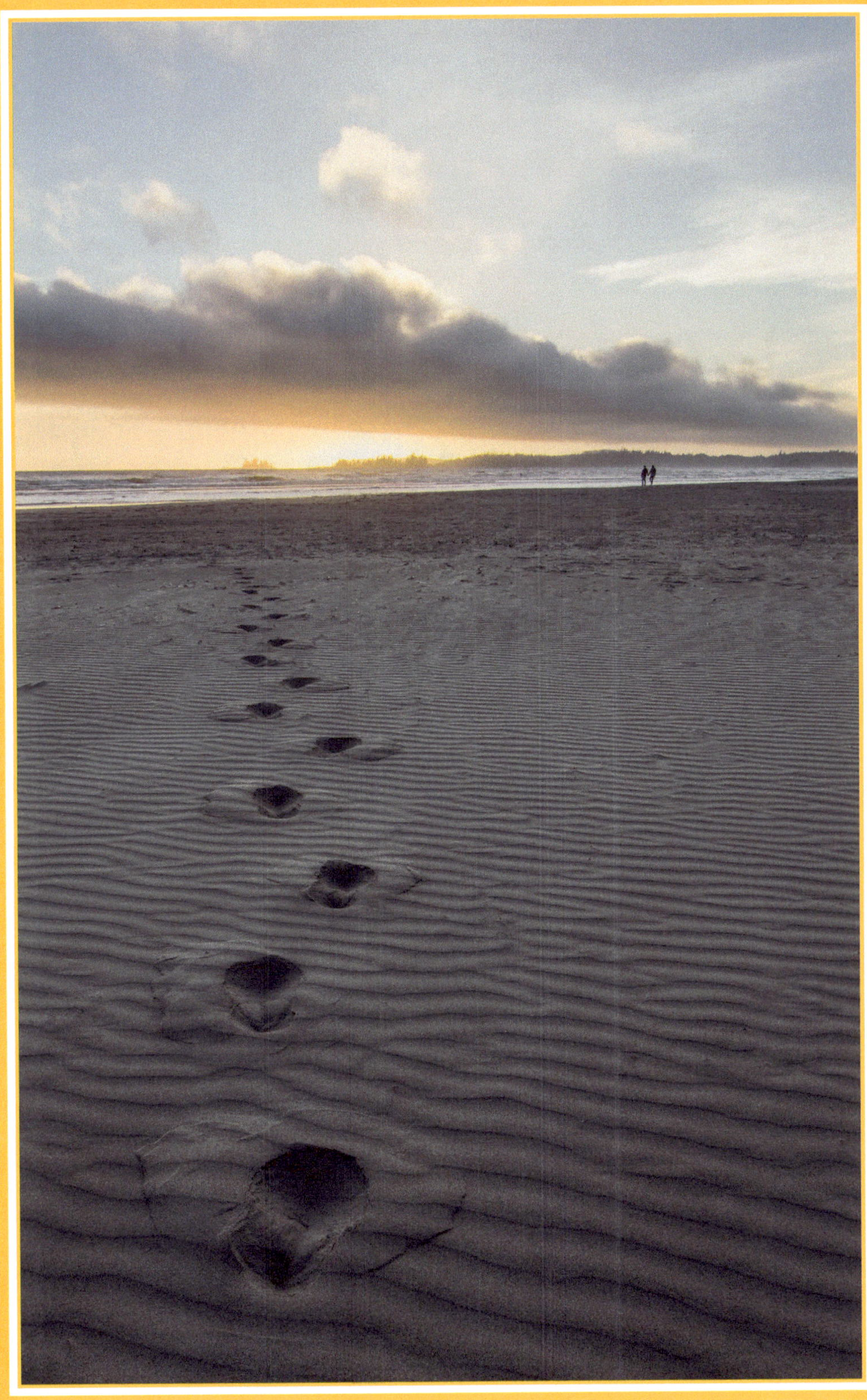

Love is patient, love is kind. It does not envy, it does not boast, it is not proud.

1 Corinthians 13:4

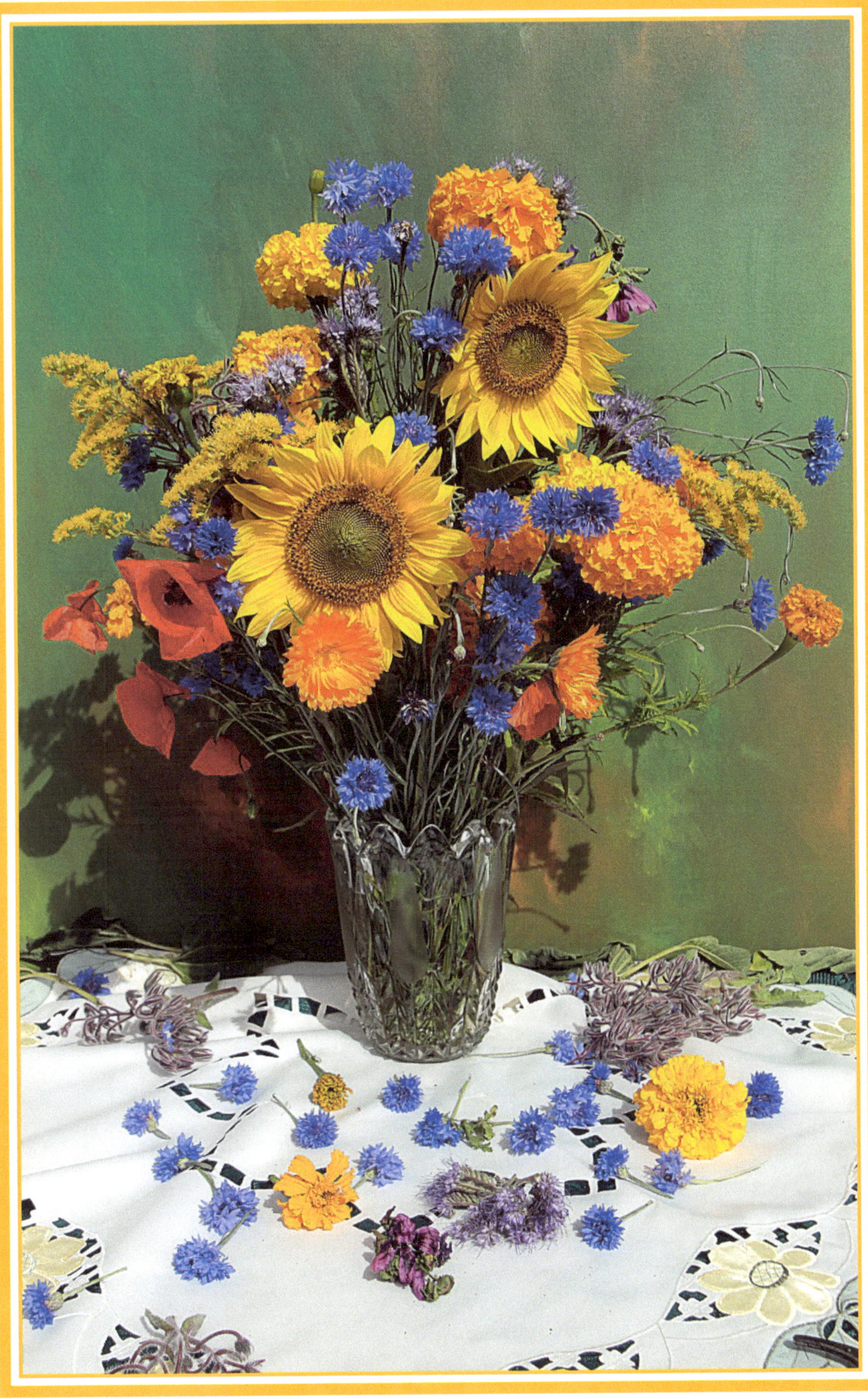

I can do all this through him who gives me strength.

Philippians 4:13

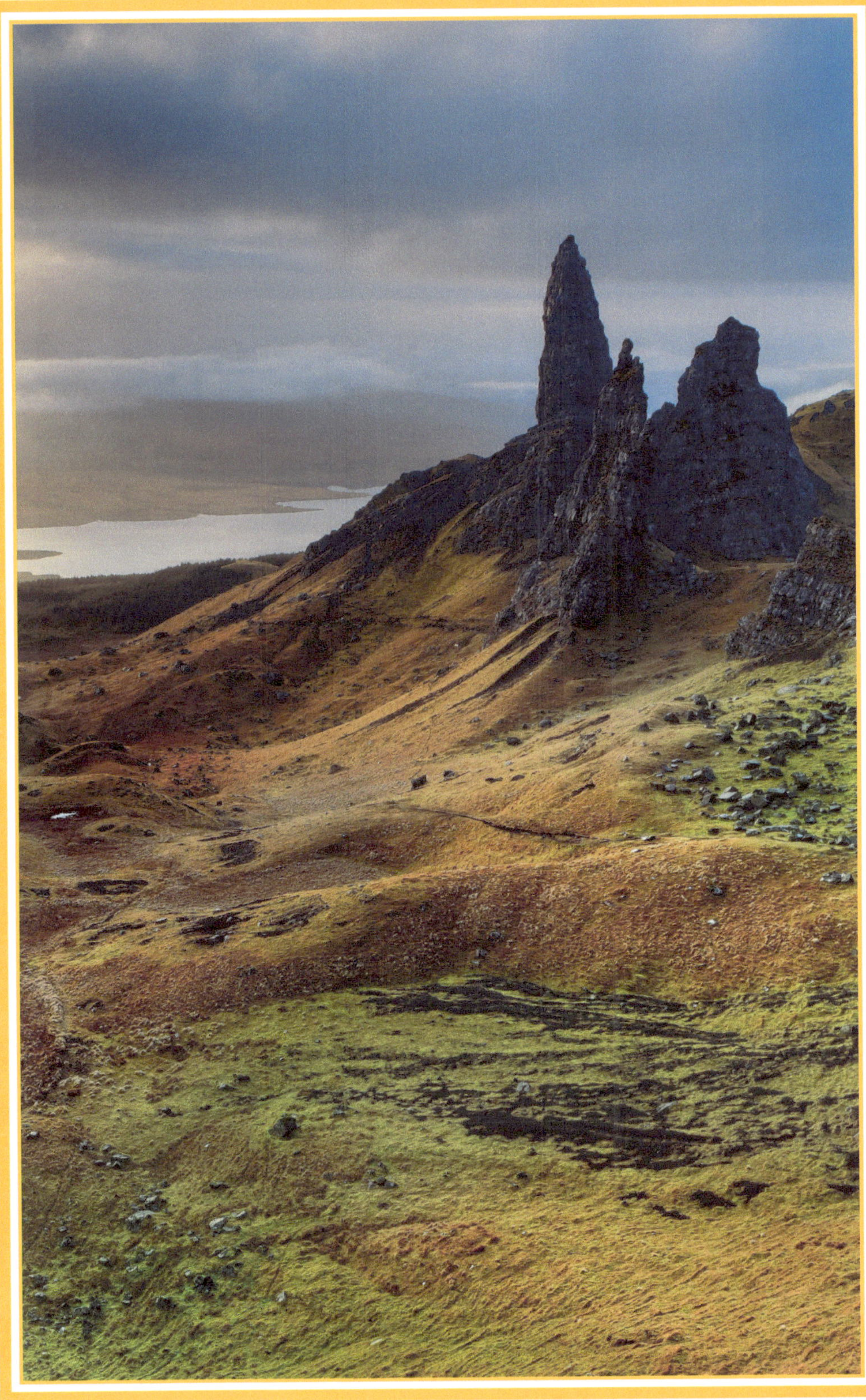

For God so loved the world that he gave his one and only Son, that whoever believes in him shall not perish but have eternal life.

John 3:16

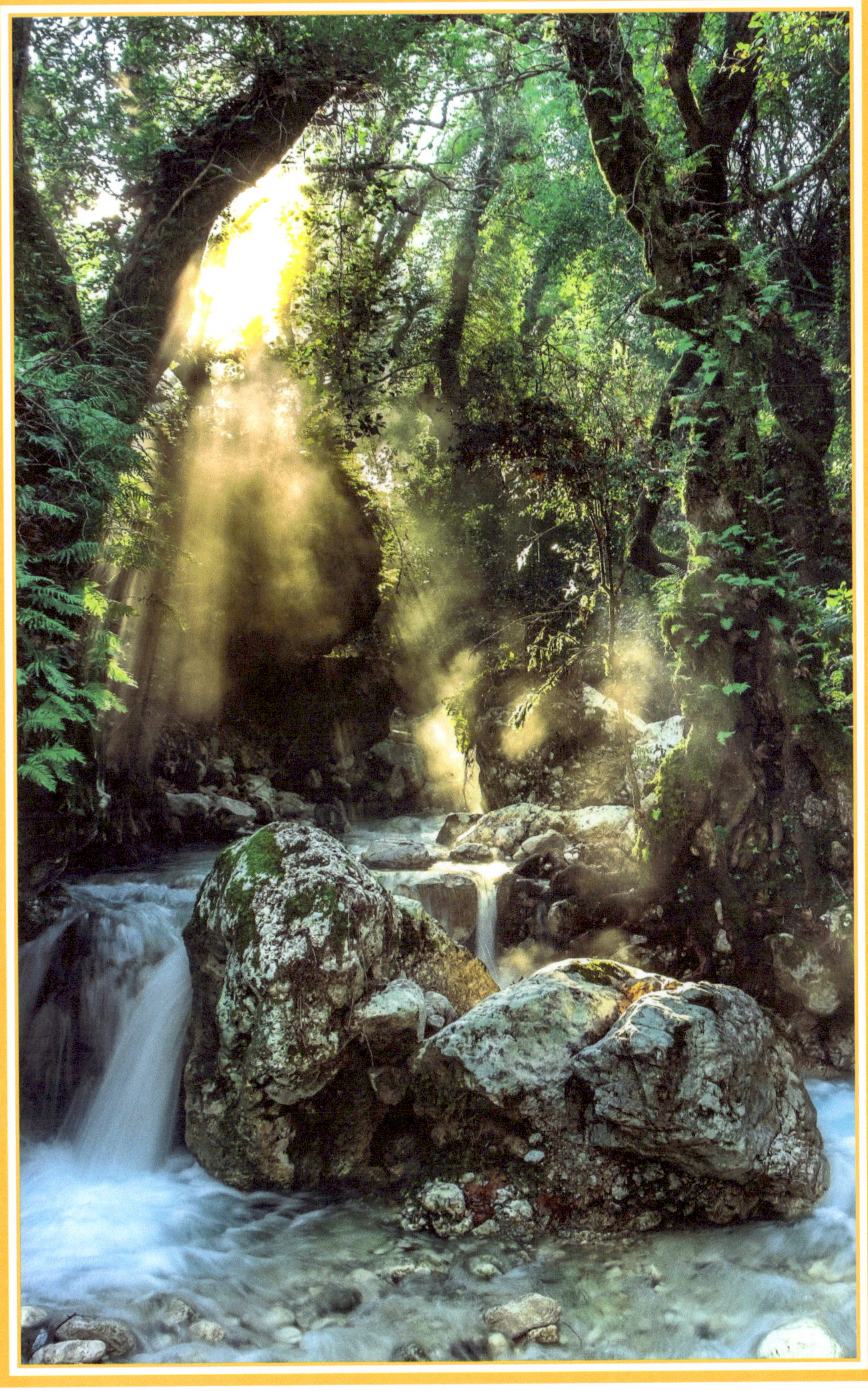

And we know that in all things God works for the good of those who love him, who have been called according to his purpose.

Romans 8:28

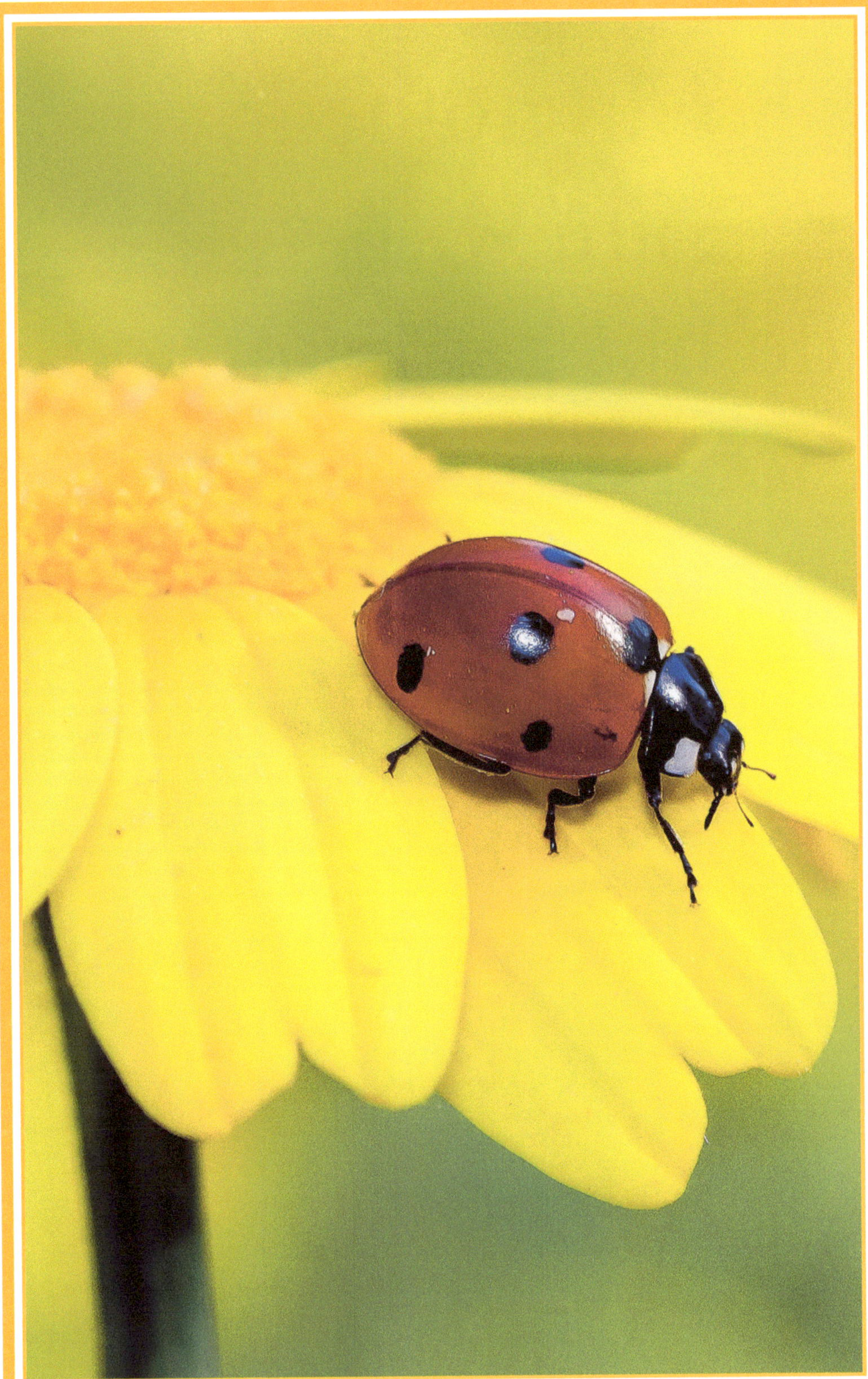

So do not fear, for
I am with you;
do not be dismayed,
for I am your God.
I will strengthen
you and help you;
I will uphold you
with my righteous
right hand.

Isaiah 41:10

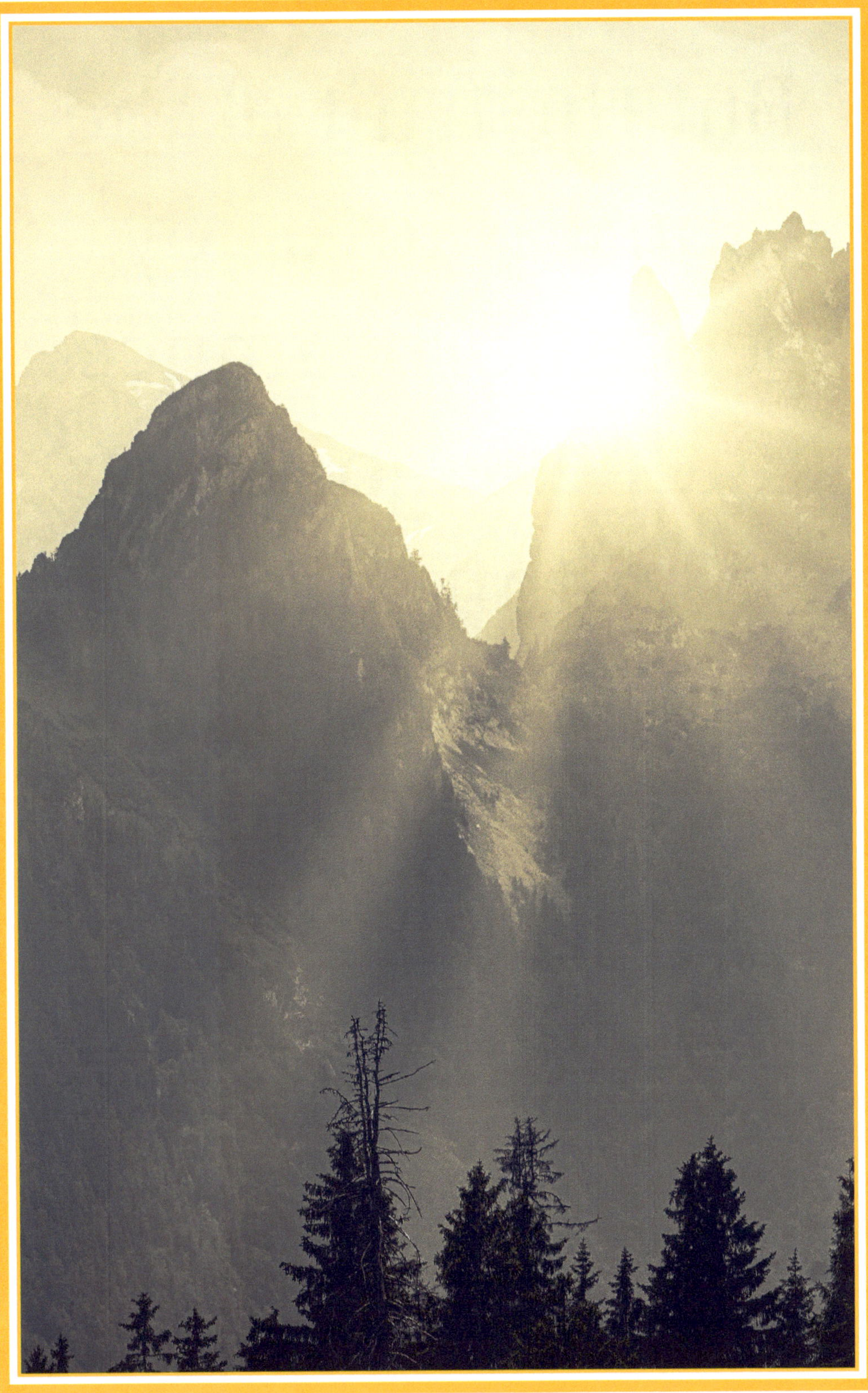

But the fruit of the spirit is love, joy, peace, forbearance, kindness, goodness, faithfulness, gentleness and self-control. Against such things there is no law.

Galatians 5:22-23

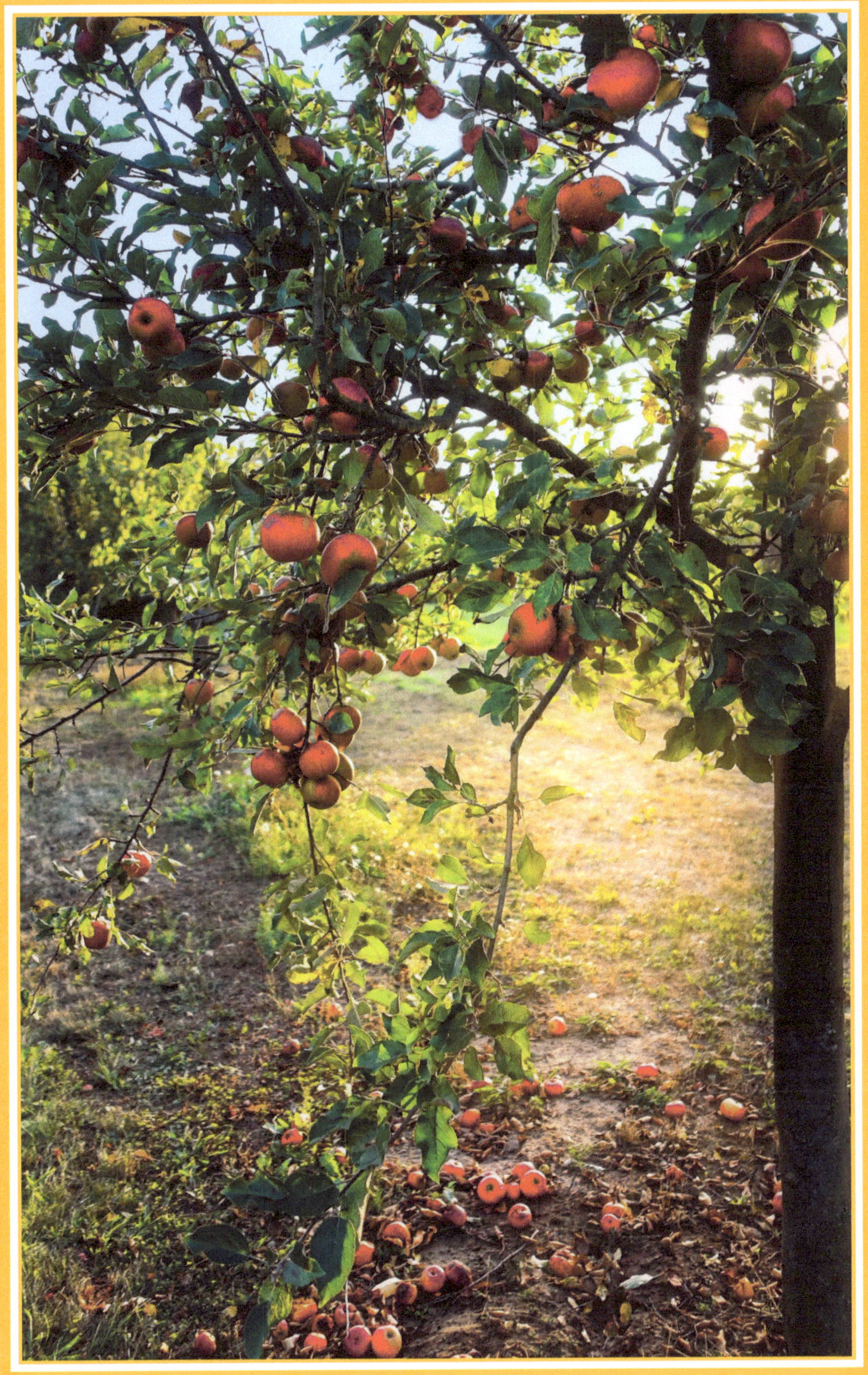

For the spirit God gave us does not make us timid, but gives us power, love and self-discipline.

2 Timothy 1:7

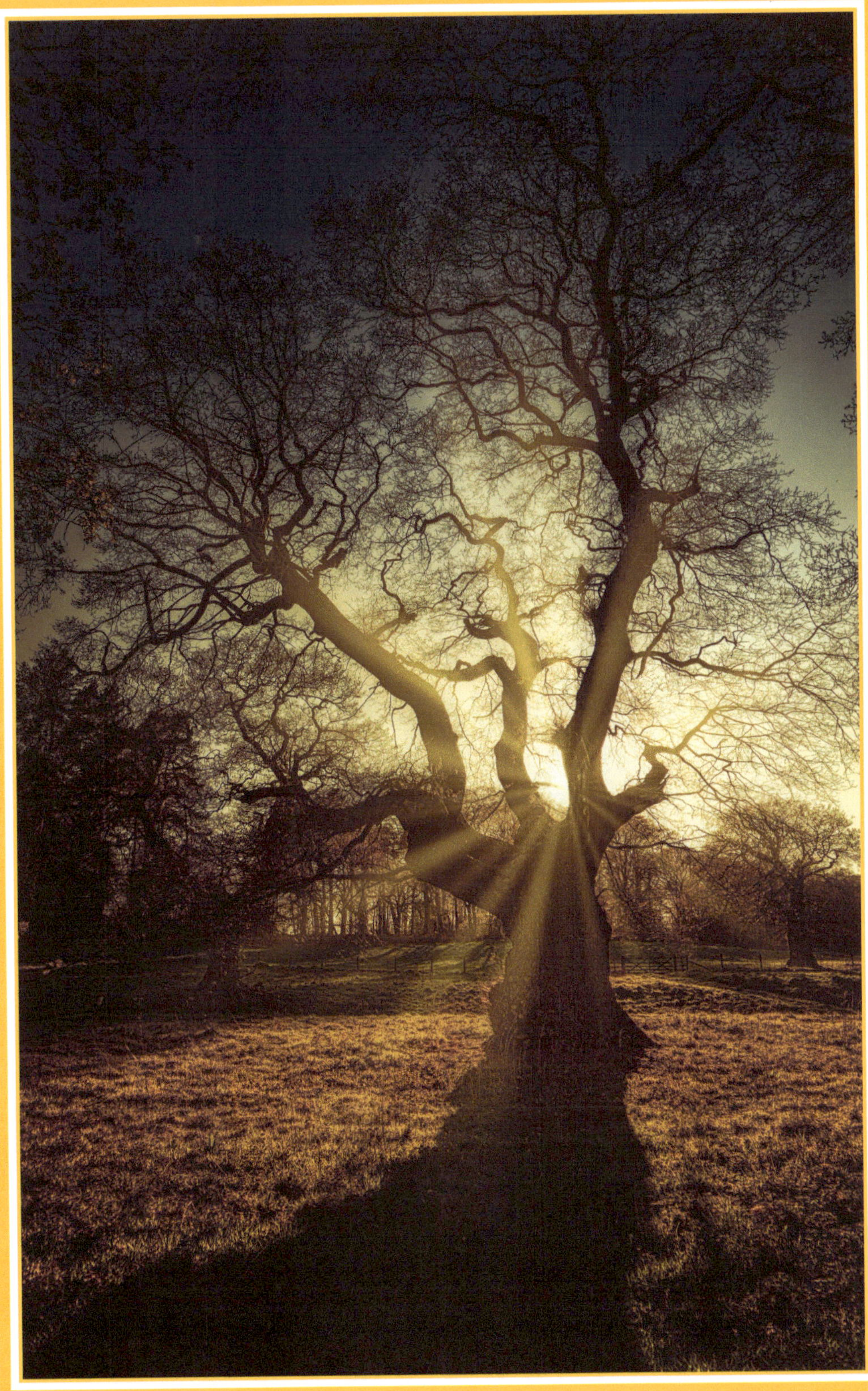

But those who hope in the LORD will renew their strength. They will soar on wings like eagles; they will run and not grow weary, they will walk and not be faint.

Isaiah 40:31

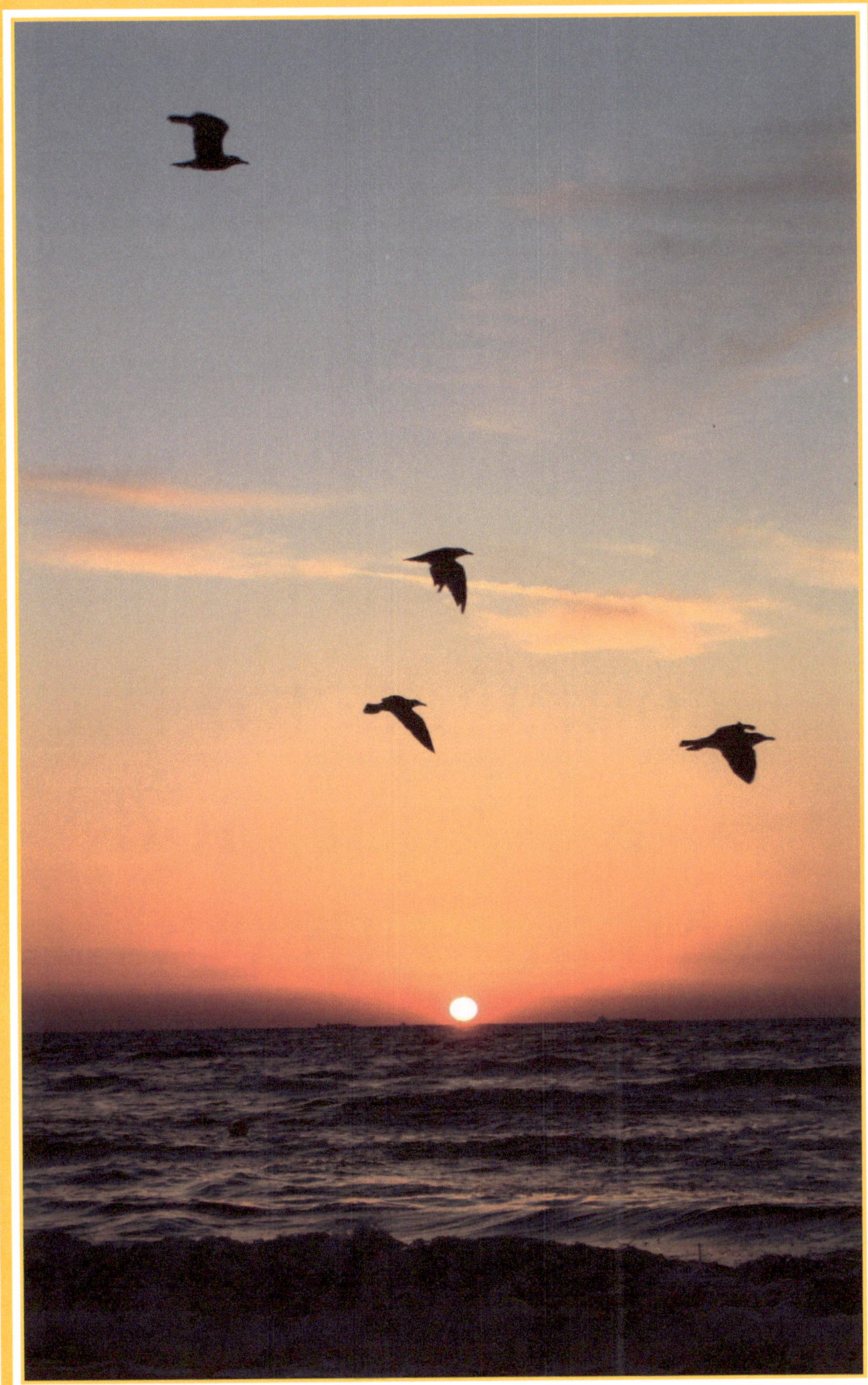

Have I not commanded you? Be strong and courageous. Do not be afraid; do not be discouraged, for the LORD your God will be with you wherever you go.

Joshua 1:9

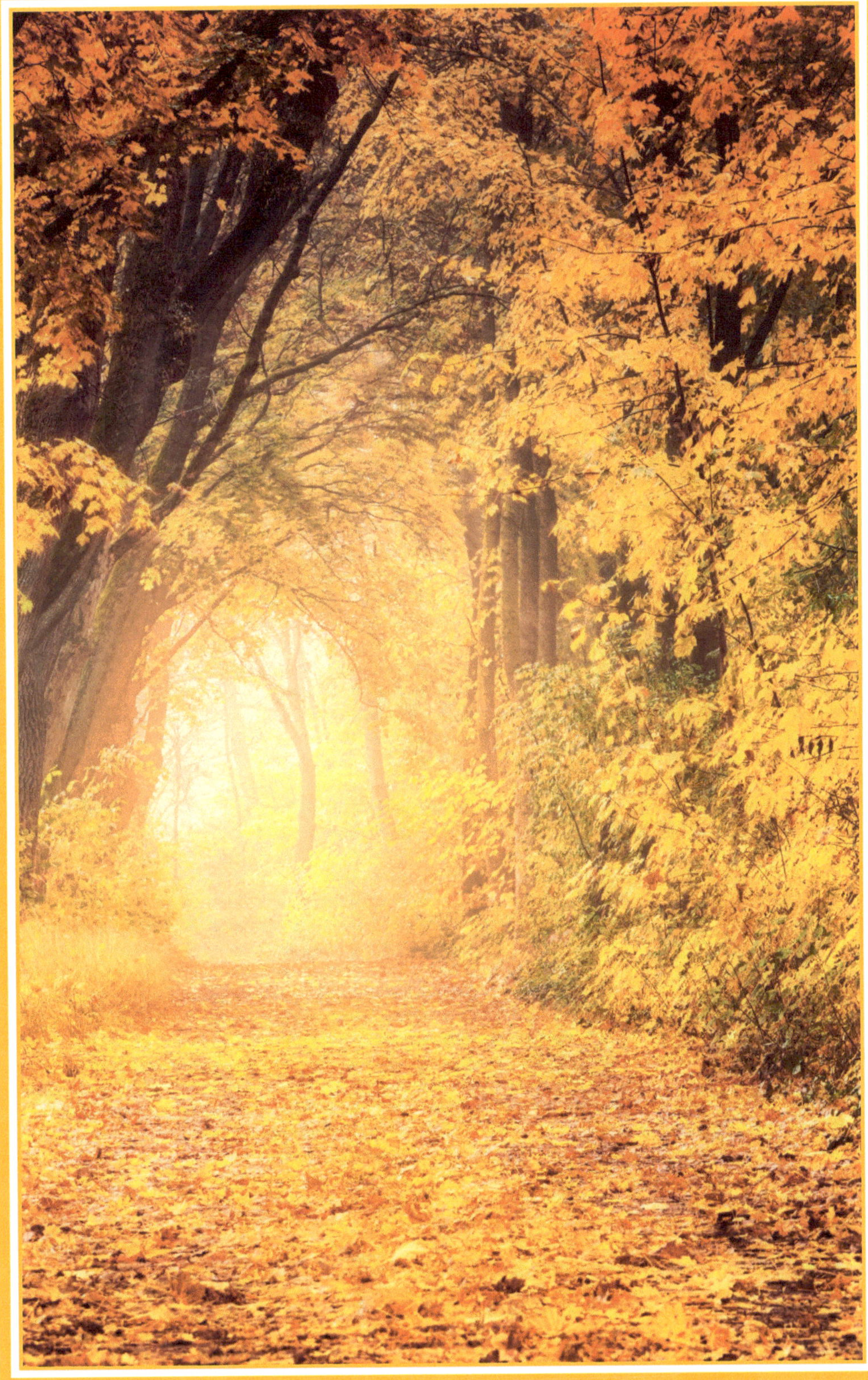

Therefore confess your sins to each other and pray for each other so that you may be healed. The prayer of a righteous person is powerful and effective.

James 5:16

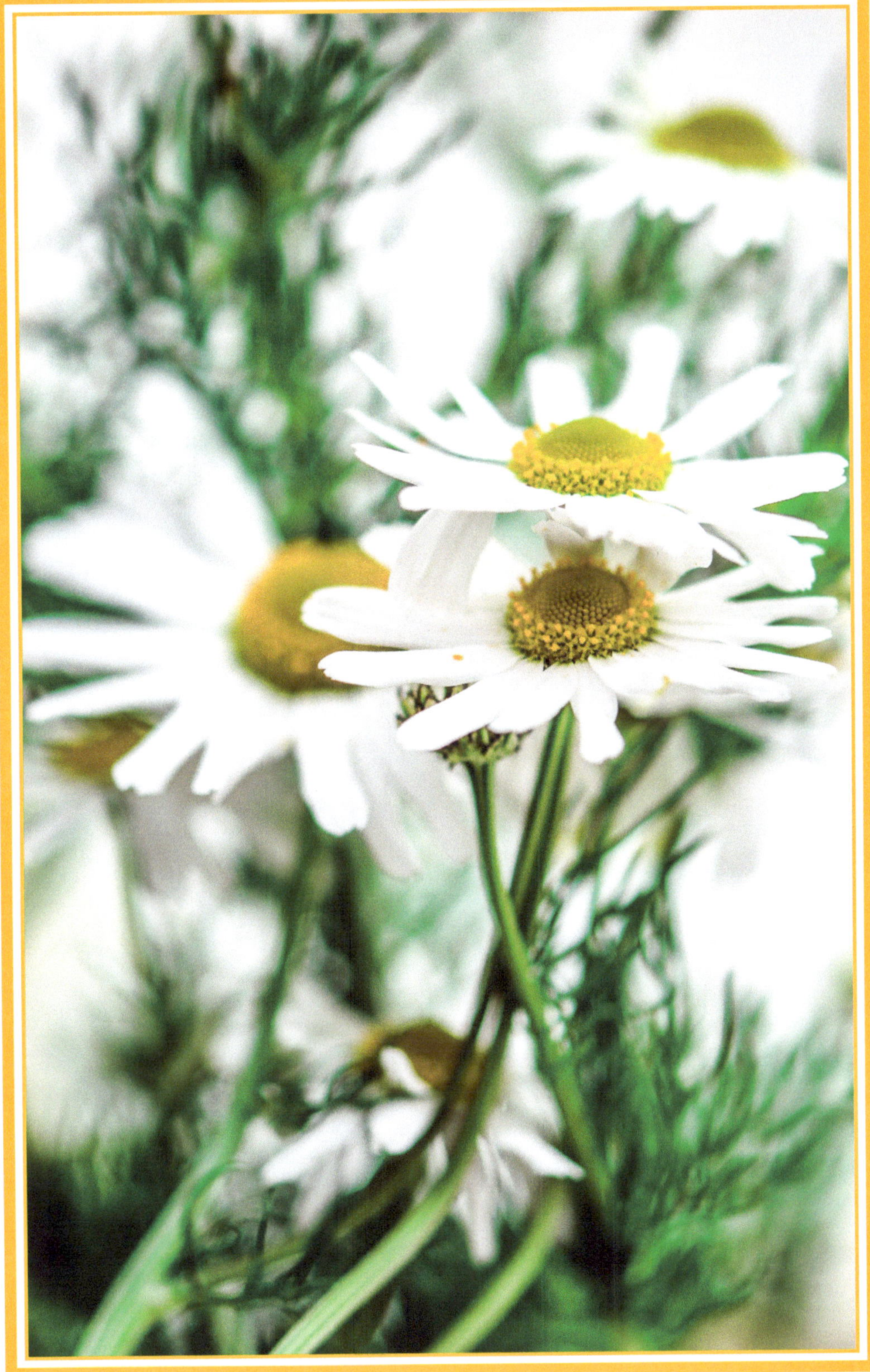

Be strong and courageous. Do not be afraid or terrified because of them, for the LORD your God goes with you; he will never leave you nor forsake you.

Deuteronomy 31:6

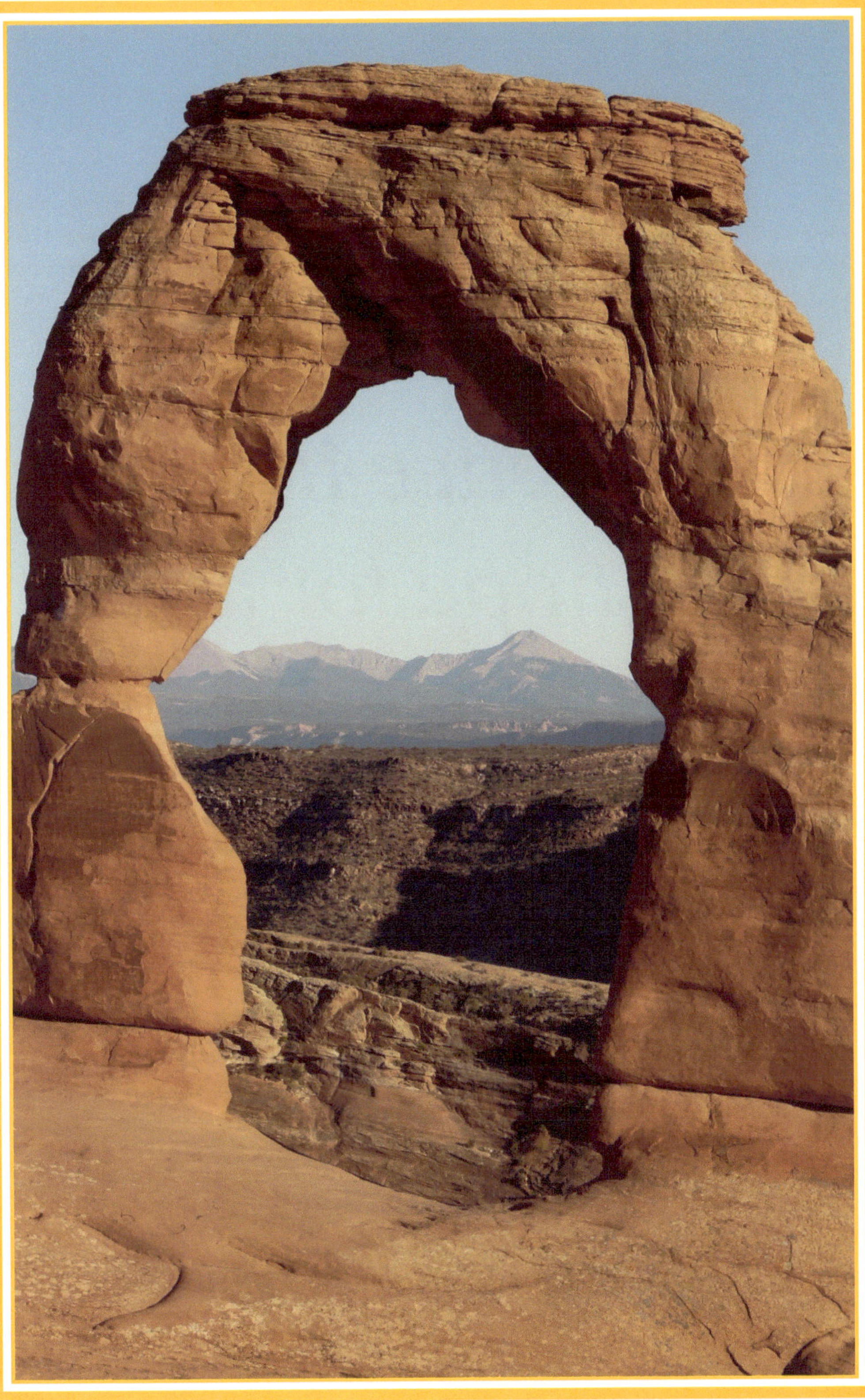

Now faith is confidence in what we hope for and assurance about what we do not see.

Hebrews 11:1

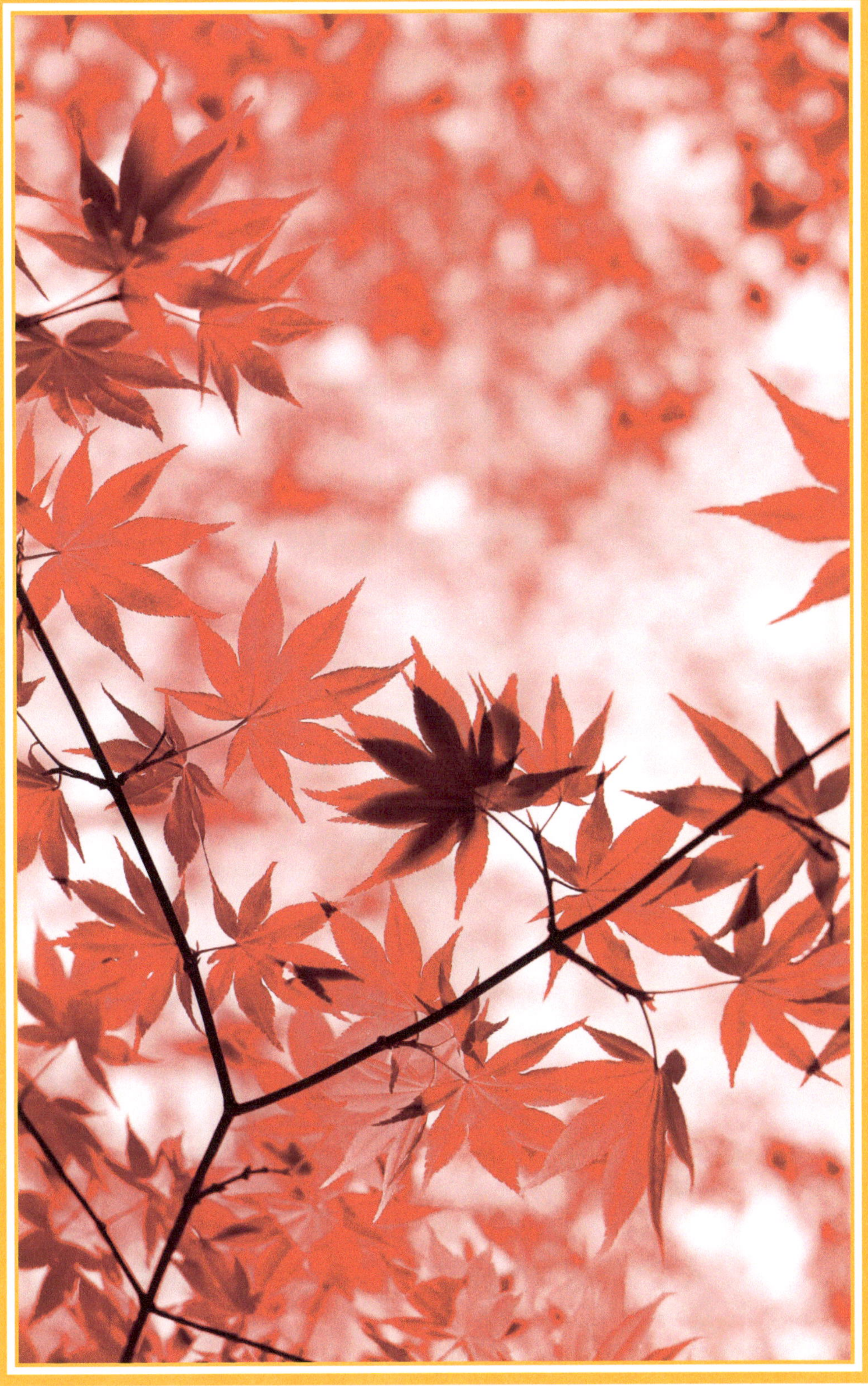

Be on your guard;
stand firm in the
faith; be courageous;
be strong.

1 Corinthians 16:13

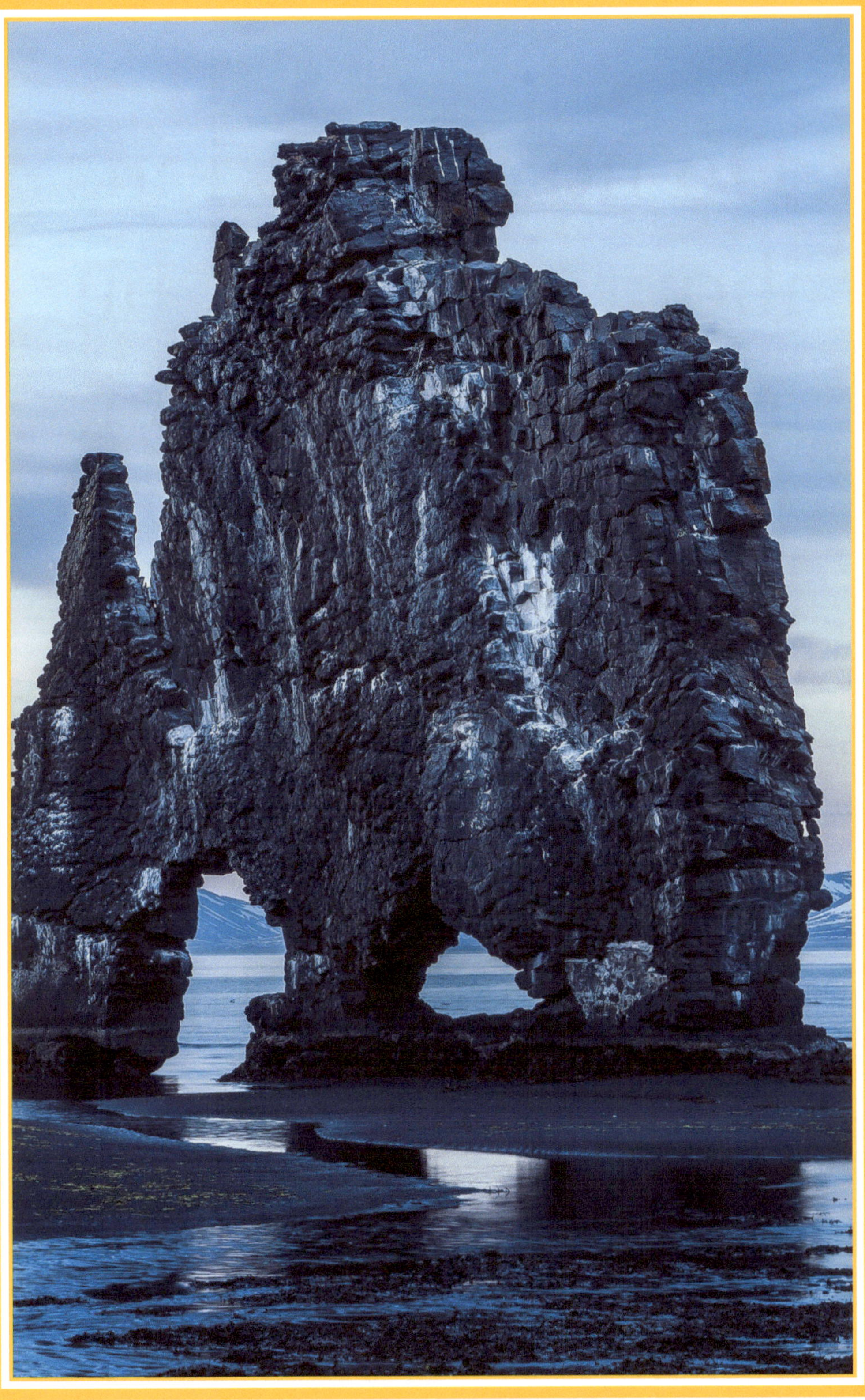

Do not be anxious
about anything, but
in every situation,
by prayer and
petition,
with thanksgiving,
present your
requests to God.

Philippians 4:6

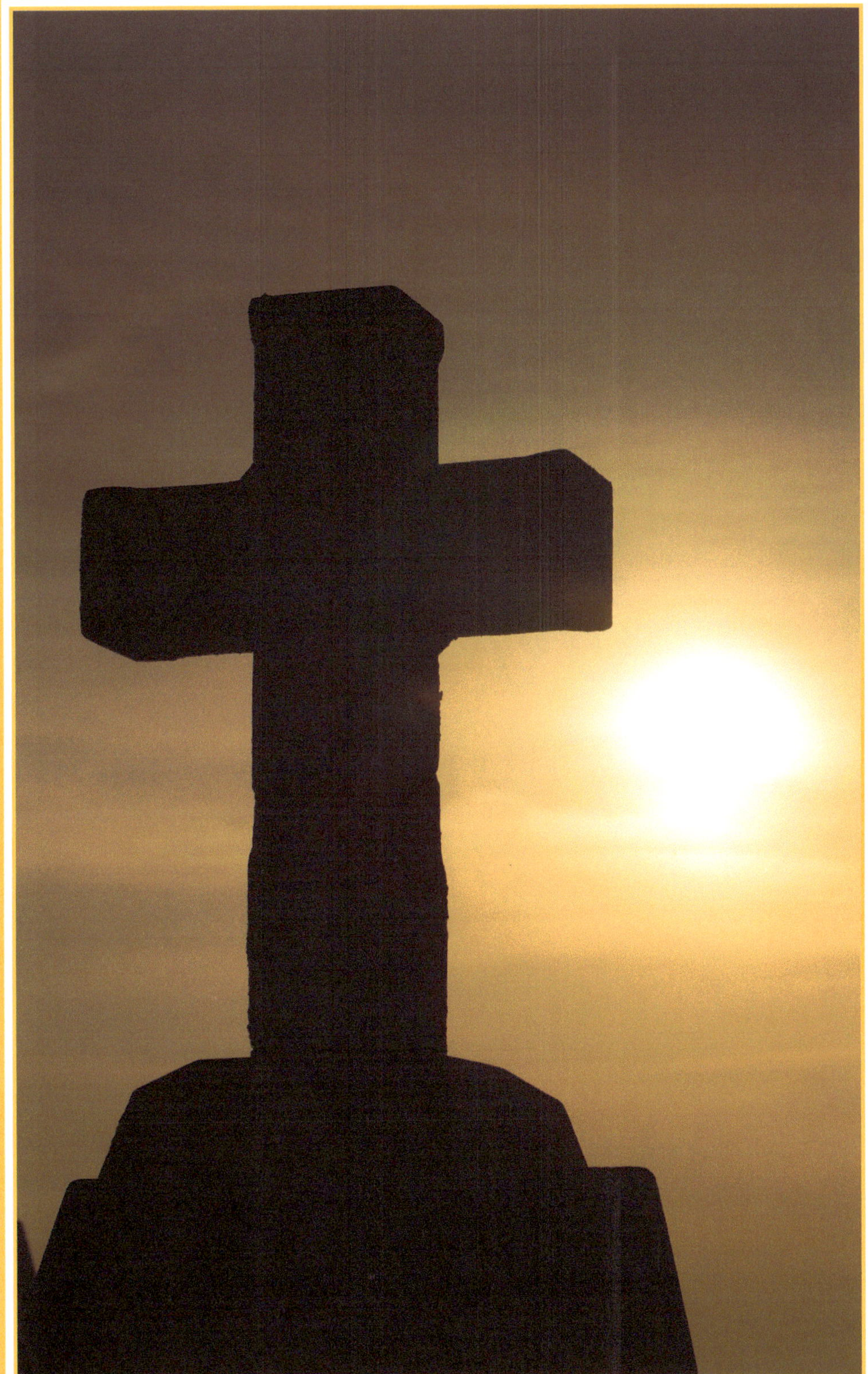

Even though I walk
through the valley
of the shadow of
death, I will fear no
evil, for you are with
me. Your rod and
your staff, they
comfort me.

Psalm 23:4

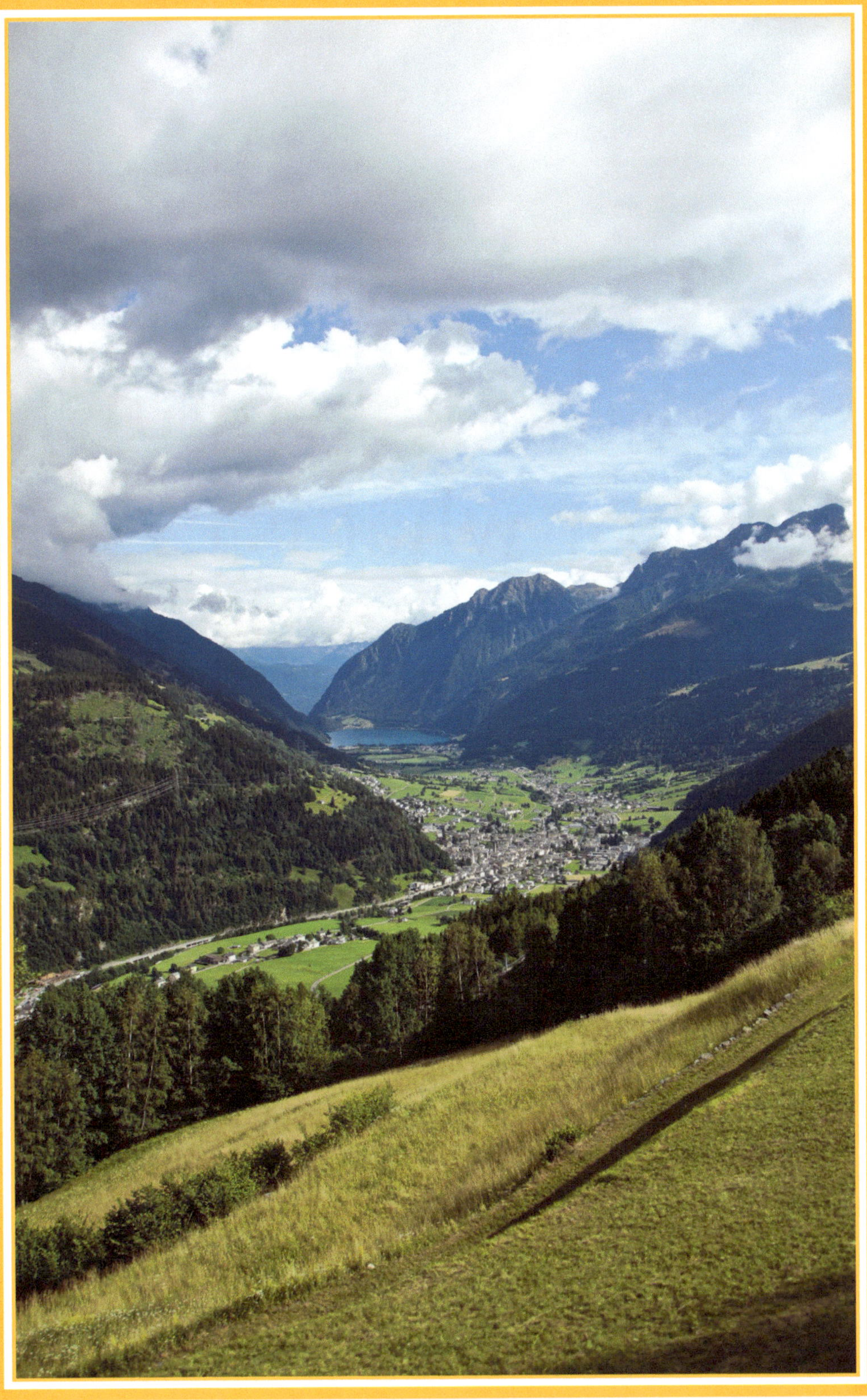

Let love be genuine.
Abhor what is evil;
hold fast to what is
good.

Romans 12:9

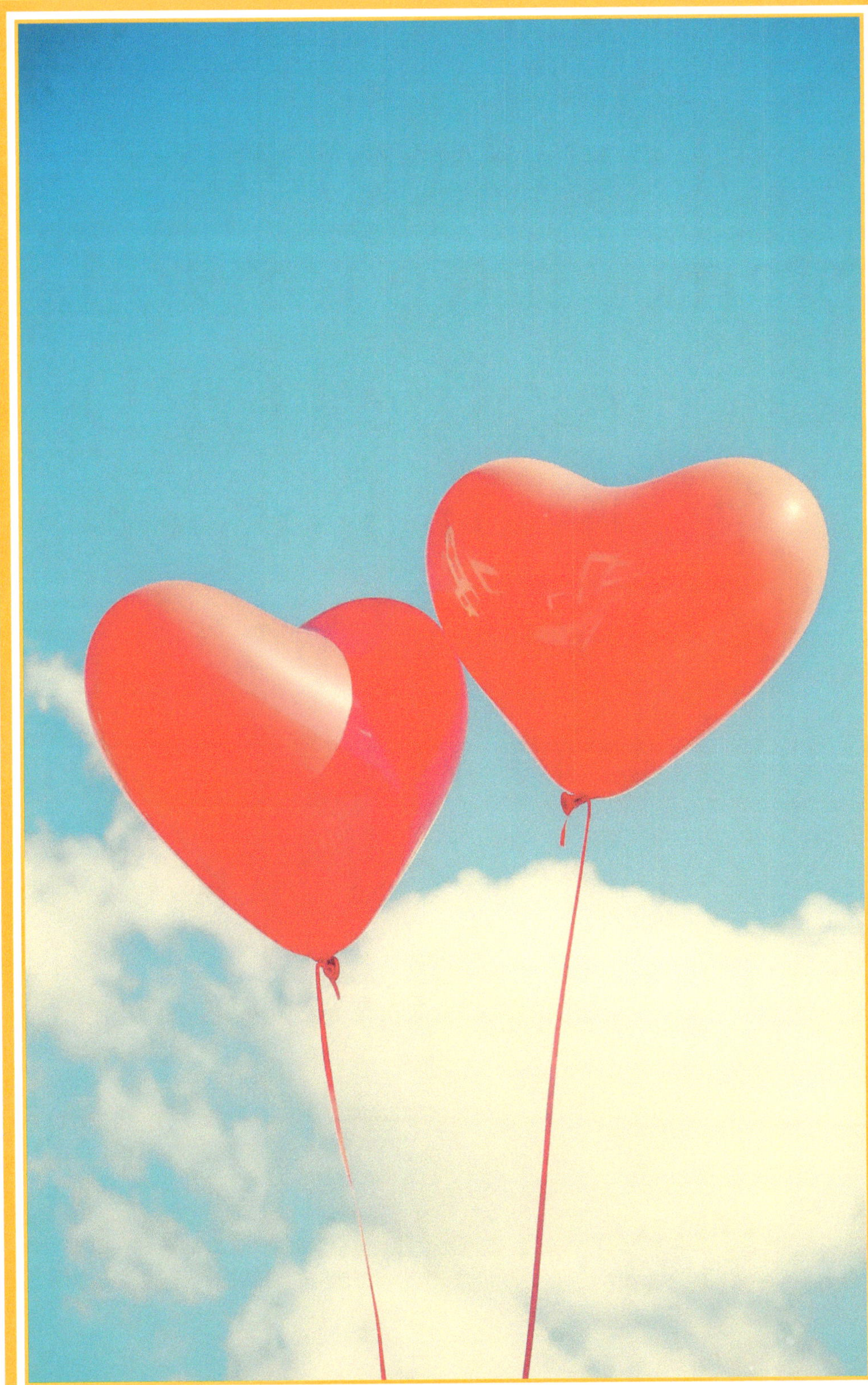

"For I know the
plans I have for you,"
declares the LORD,
"plans to prosper
you and not
to harm you, plans
to give you hope
and a future.

Jeremiah 29:11

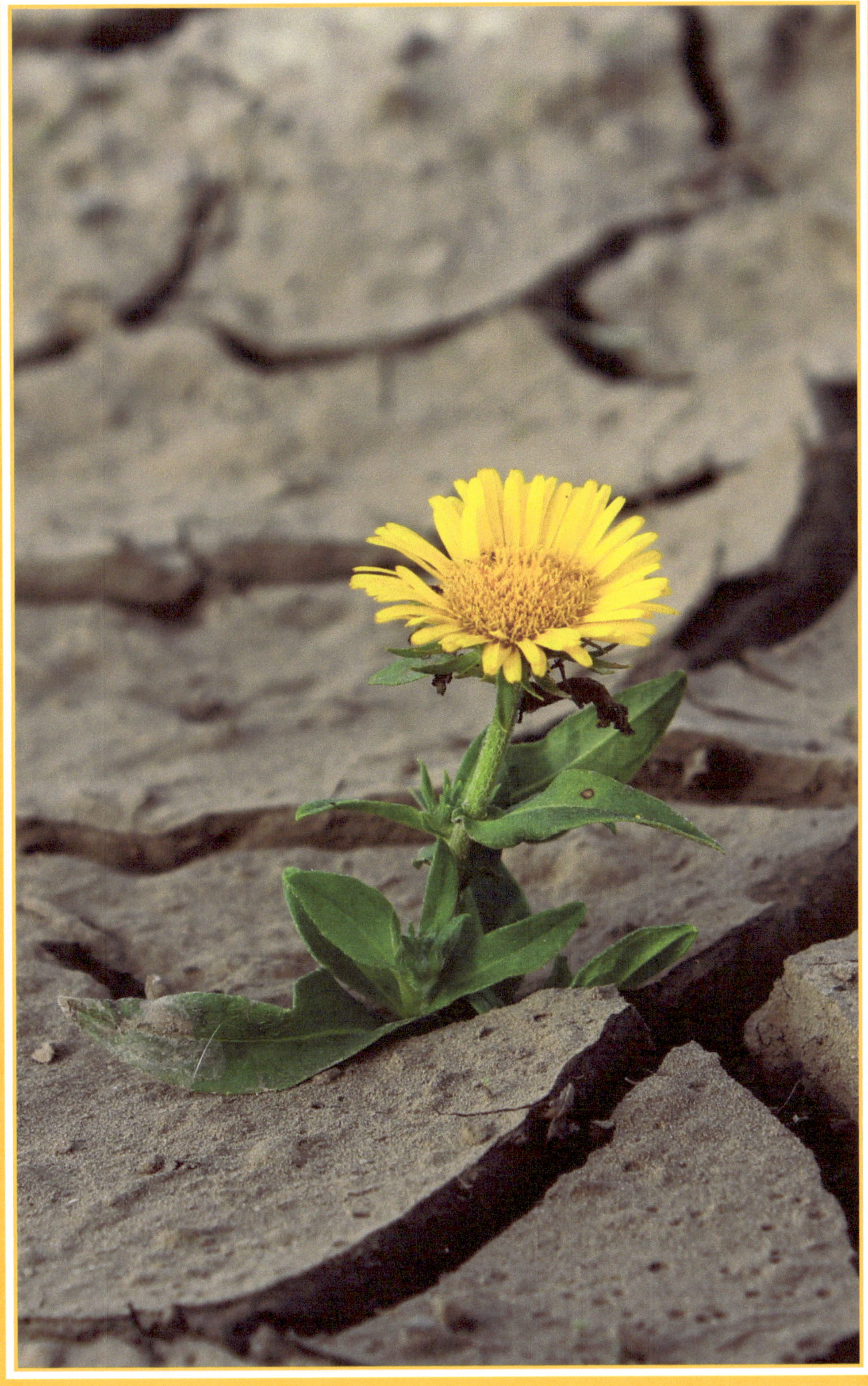

Cast all your
anxiety on him
because he
cares for you.

1 Peter 5:7

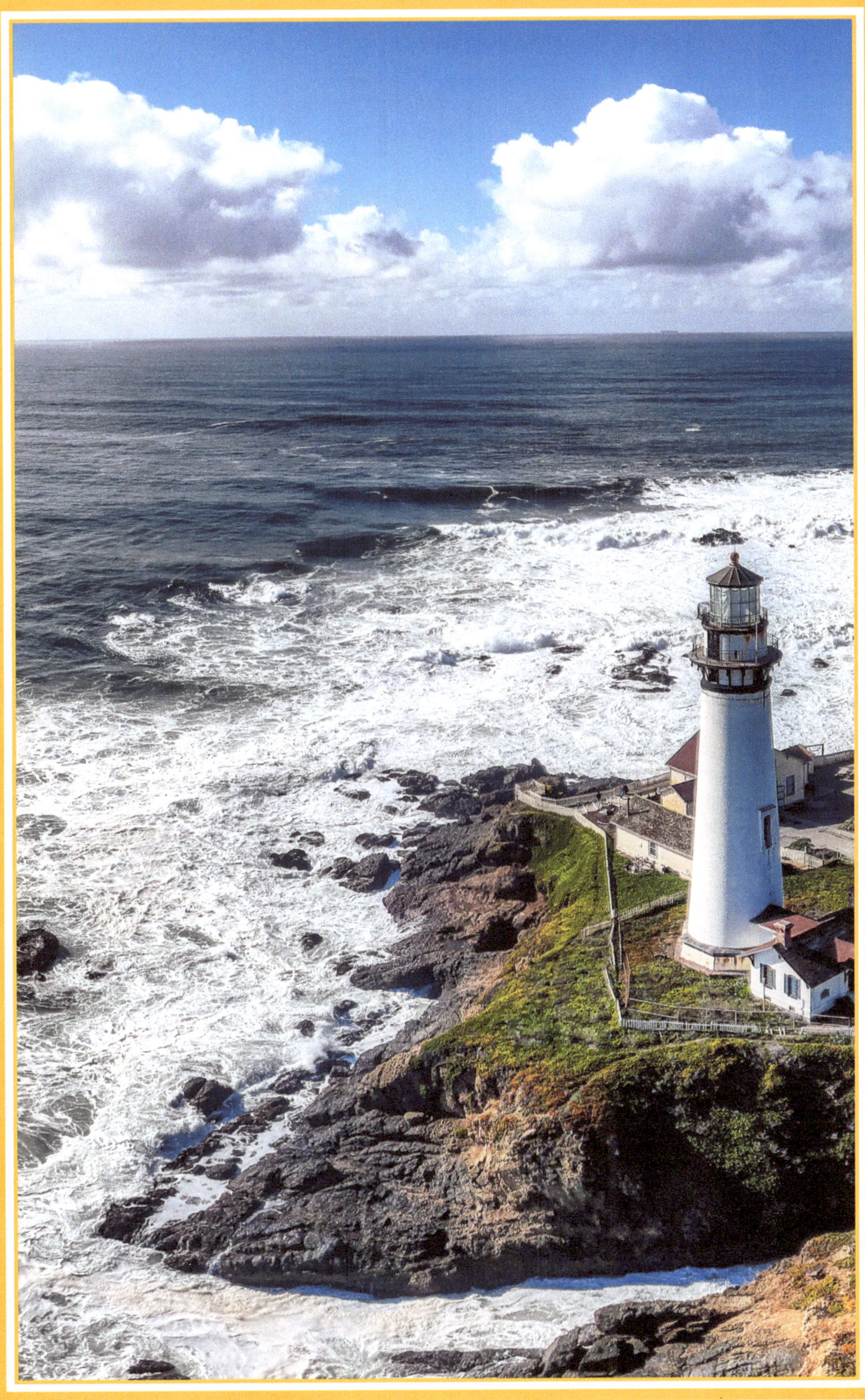

The LORD your God is with you, the Mighty Warrior who saves. He will take great delight in you; in his love he will no longer rebuke you, but will rejoice over you with singing.

Zephaniah 3:17

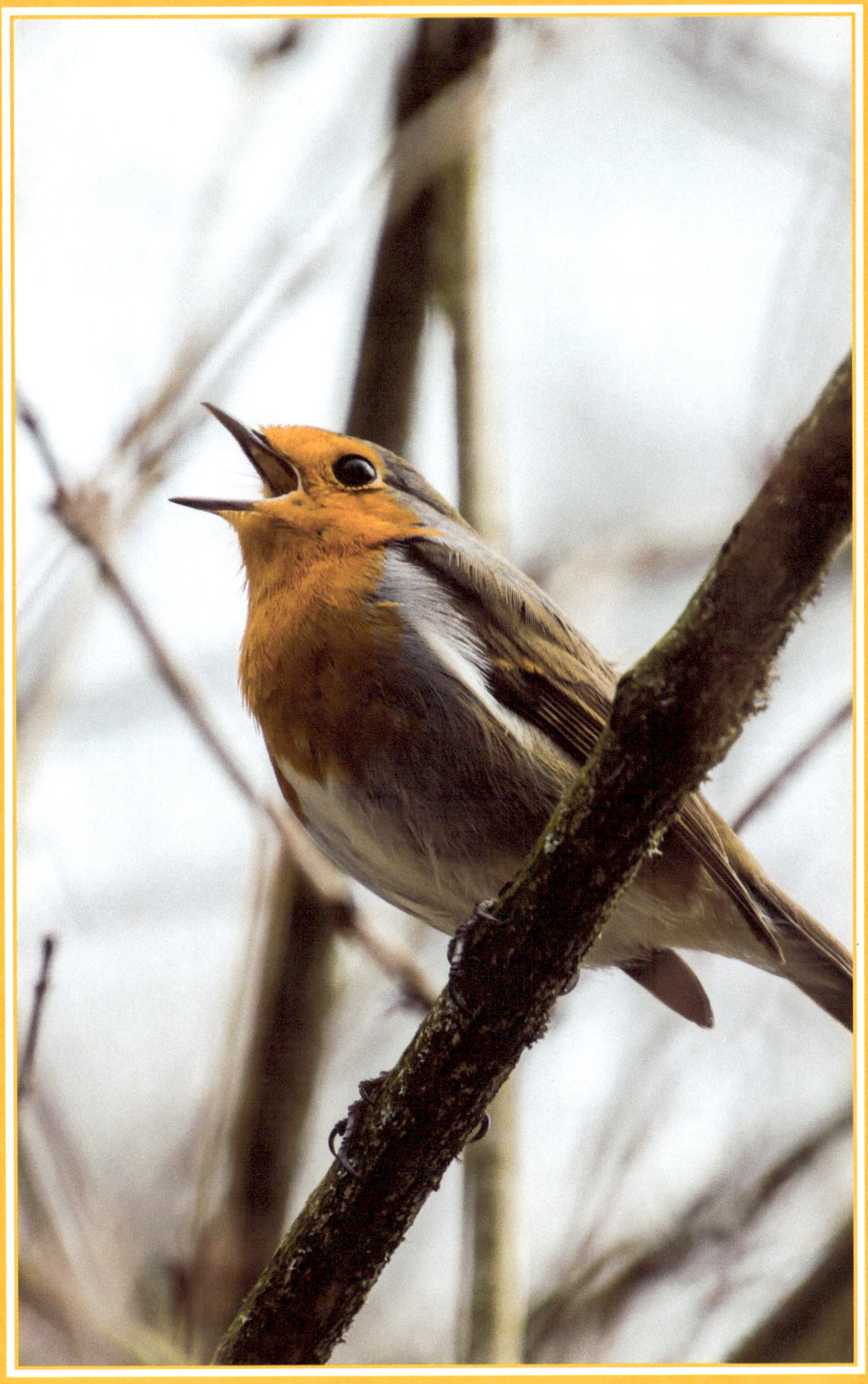